NO GALLBLADDER DIET COOKBOOK FOR WOMEN

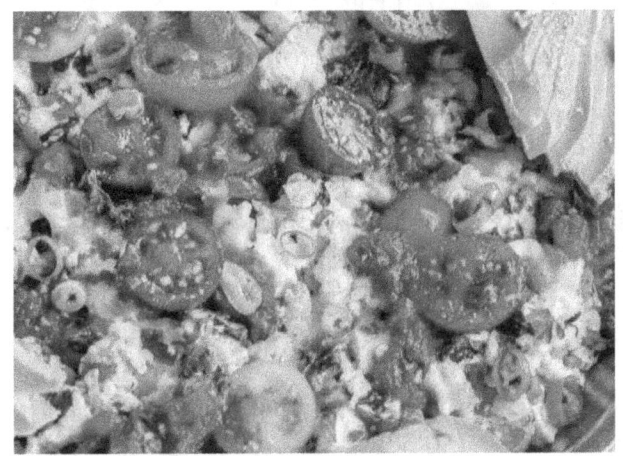

The Ultimate Guide to Flavorful and Delicious Recipes to Revitalize Your Metabolism After Gallbladder Removal, With 30 Day Meal Plan.

Sharon D. Stacy

Table of Contents

SCAN THIS CODE TO GAIN ACCESS TO MORE BOOKS BY THE AUTHOR

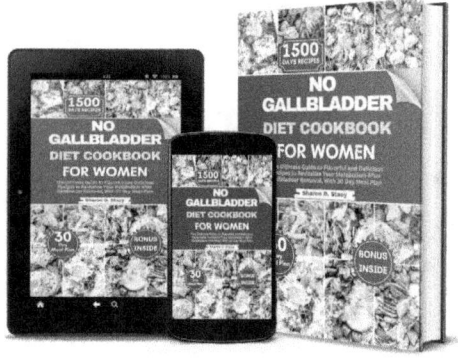

How to Use This Book

1. Introduction: Begin by reading the introduction and gain insight into the importance of a gallbladder-friendly diet for women. Understand the functions of the gallbladder, common issues post-surgery, and foods to avoid.

2. No Gallbladder Lifestyle For Women: Understand the healthy lifestyle tips for women adapting to life without a gallbladder ranging from their diets, exercise, stress management etc.

3. Meal Planning: Explore the 30-day meal plan provided, which offers a diverse range of breakfast, lunch, dinner, and snack options. Use this plan as a guide to structure your meals for optimal nutrition and variety.

4. Recipes: Browse through the breakfast, lunch, dinner, and snack recipes, each meticulously crafted with women's health in mind. Ingredients, preparation methods, nutritional value, and cooking times are clearly outlined for easy reference.

5. Shopping List: Refer to the comprehensive shopping list provided to ensure you have all the necessary ingredients on hand. Organized by category, this list simplifies the grocery shopping process and helps you stay organized.

6. Meal Planner Journal: Utilize the meal planner journal section to customize your meal plans and track your progress. Write down your weekly menus, jot down any notes or modifications, and reflect on how each meal makes you feel.

7. Notes/Progress Report: Take advantage of the notes and progress report section to document your journey. Record any changes in your symptoms, energy levels, or overall well-being as you follow the diet.

8. Special Motivation: Finally, remember the special motivation provided in the conclusion. Let it serve as a reminder of your commitment to your health and wellness journey. Embrace each recipe with enthusiasm and dedication, knowing that you are taking proactive steps towards a healthier and happier life.

By following these steps and embracing the resources provided in the "No Gallbladder Diet Cookbook for Women", you'll be well-equipped to embark on your journey towards better health and vitality.

Enjoy the delicious recipes, nourish your body with wholesome ingredients, and savor the satisfaction of knowing that you are prioritizing your well-being.

INTRODUCTION

Are you fed up with having your food restricted because of gallbladder problems? Do you ever find yourself questioning whether there's a way to eat tasty food without having to worry about discomfort or digestive issues? You are not alone. After having surgery to remove their gallbladder, many women experience similar difficulties, and looking for dietary remedies can be daunting. However, what if I told you that the common knowledge about diets following gallbladder surgery could not be totally true?

Many think that following a bland, low-fat diet is the best way to live without a gallbladder. Although at first this technique seems reasonable, it ignores the complexity of the problem and is based on outdated information. It's a fact that a one-size-fits-all approach to post-gallbladder surgery nutrition ignores the unique requirements and preferences of every woman.

Living without a gallbladder can bring with it certain difficulties, but it also makes cooking new foods possible. Just imagine enjoying tasty meals without having to worry about pain or digestive issues. What if you could enjoy the flavors and ingredients you love without sacrificing the health of your digestive system?

You're going to embark on a journey of culinary exploration and empowerment with the help of the "No Gallbladder Diet Cookbook For Women." This book offers a full guidance on taking back control of your nutrition and life, not just a list of recipes. Within are a plethora of resources on gallbladder health, nutrient-dense foods, and delectable recipes designed especially for women adjusting to life without a gallbladder.

As a professional nutritionist, I understand the frustration and uncertainty that can accompany gallbladder issues. For this reason, I've poured my knowledge and love into this cookbook, providing you useful tips and delectable dishes that will fuel your body and spirit. A world of culinary delights awaits you when you bid farewell to bland, restrictive diets. With the "No Gallbladder Diet Cookbook For Women" by your side, you'll discover how to enjoy food again with confidence and joy.

CHAPTER 1

What is Gallbladder?

The gallbladder is a small, pear-shaped organ located beneath the liver in the upper right abdomen. Its primary function is to store and concentrate bile, a digestive fluid produced by the liver. When food is consumed, especially fatty foods, the gallbladder contracts and releases bile into the small intestine to aid in the digestion and absorption of fats and fat-soluble vitamins.

Bile, which is composed of water, cholesterol, bile salts, bilirubin, and other substances, helps emulsify fats, breaking them down into smaller particles that can be more easily digested by enzymes in the small intestine. This process allows the body to absorb essential nutrients from food, such as vitamins A, D, E, and K.

In addition to storing and concentrating bile, the gallbladder also plays a role in regulating the flow of bile into the small intestine. The release of bile is controlled by hormones and nerve signals triggered by the presence of food in the digestive tract.

While the gallbladder serves an important function in the digestive process, it is not considered essential for survival. In cases where the gallbladder becomes diseased or dysfunctional, such as in the presence of gallstones, gallbladder inflammation (cholecystitis), or other gallbladder disorders, surgical removal of the gallbladder, known as cholecystectomy, may be necessary to alleviate symptoms and prevent complications.

The gallbladder is a vital organ that plays a key role in digestion, particularly in the breakdown and absorption of dietary fats. Its proper functioning is essential for maintaining digestive health and overall well-being.

Functions of Gallbladder

The gallbladder is a small but essential organ in the digestive system, primarily responsible for storing and concentrating bile produced by the liver. Here are the primary functions of the gallbladder, they include:

1.   Bile Storage: The primary function of the gallbladder is to store bile, a digestive fluid produced by the liver. Between meals, bile accumulates and becomes concentrated in the gallbladder, making it more potent and effective in aiding digestion when released into the small intestine during meals.

2.   Bile Concentration: In addition to storing bile, the gallbladder concentrates it by removing water and electrolytes. This process helps to increase the potency of bile, ensuring that it is

highly effective in emulsifying fats and aiding in their digestion.

3.   **Bile Release:** When food, especially fatty foods, enters the small intestine, signals are sent to the gallbladder to contract and release bile into the duodenum (the first part of the small intestine). The bile helps emulsify fats, breaking them down into smaller droplets that can be more easily digested by enzymes and absorbed by the intestinal lining.

4.   **Facilitating Nutrient Absorption:** Bile plays a crucial role in the absorption of fats and fat-soluble vitamins (such as vitamins A, D, E, and K) from the small intestine into the bloodstream. By emulsifying fats, bile enables them to be more readily absorbed by the intestinal cells and transported throughout the body.

5.   **Regulation of Bile Flow:** The gallbladder helps regulate the flow of bile into the small intestine, ensuring that bile is released in

appropriate amounts in response to the presence of food. Hormonal and neural signals trigger the gallbladder to contract and release bile when needed for digestion.

The gallbladder's functions are essential for efficient digestion and nutrient absorption, particularly in the breakdown and utilization of dietary fats. While it is possible to live without a gallbladder, its proper functioning significantly contributes to overall digestive health and well-being.

Common Issues After Gallbladder Removal in Women

After gallbladder removal surgery, also known as cholecystectomy, women may experience a variety of common issues as their bodies adjust to the absence of the gallbladder. These issues can vary in severity and duration from person to person. Some of the most common issues experienced by women after gallbladder removal include:

1.   **Digestive Symptoms:** Many women experience digestive symptoms such as diarrhea, bloating, gas, and abdominal discomfort, particularly after consuming fatty or greasy foods. This is often due to the absence of the gallbladder, which previously stored and released bile to aid in fat digestion.

2.   **Postcholecystectomy Syndrome (PCS):** Some women may develop postcholecystectomy

syndrome, which refers to persistent abdominal pain, bloating, or indigestion after gallbladder removal. This can occur due to various factors, including bile reflux, sphincter of Oddi dysfunction, or gastrointestinal disorders.

3.   **Changes in Bowel Habits:** Without the gallbladder's ability to regulate bile release, some women may experience changes in bowel habits, such as increased frequency of bowel movements or loose stools. This can occur due to excess bile entering the intestine more rapidly than it can be absorbed.

4.   **Difficulty Digesting Fatty Foods:** Since the gallbladder's primary function is to store and release bile for fat digestion, some women may have difficulty digesting fatty foods after gallbladder removal. This can lead to symptoms such as nausea, bloating, or abdominal pain after consuming high-fat meals.

5.   **Nutritional Deficiencies:** In some cases, gallbladder removal may affect the absorption of fat-soluble vitamins (such as vitamins A, D, E, and K) and essential fatty acids, leading to potential nutritional deficiencies over time. Women may need to monitor their nutrient intake and consider supplementation if deficiencies occur.

6.   **Weight Changes:** Some women may experience weight changes after gallbladder removal, either due to changes in dietary habits, alterations in fat absorption and metabolism, or fluctuations in digestive symptoms that affect appetite and calorie intake.

7.   **Gallstone Formation in the Bile Ducts:** Although rare, gallstones can still form in the bile ducts after gallbladder removal. These stones may cause symptoms such as abdominal pain, jaundice, or pancreatitis and may require further medical intervention.

It's essential for women experiencing any of these issues after gallbladder removal to consult with their healthcare provider for proper evaluation and management. Dietary modifications, lifestyle changes, and medications may help alleviate symptoms and improve quality of life post-surgery.

Gallbladder Post Surgical Diet For Women

Following gallbladder removal surgery, women may benefit from adopting a post-surgical diet that supports digestion and minimizes discomfort. While individual dietary needs may vary, here are some general guidelines for a gallbladder post-surgical diet for women:

1.   **Gradual Introduction of Foods:** Initially, start with a bland and low-fat diet, gradually reintroducing foods as tolerated. Begin with easily digestible foods such as broth-based soups, cooked vegetables, lean proteins, and whole grains.

2.   **Limit Fatty and Fried Foods:** Avoid or limit high-fat and fried foods, as they can be difficult to digest without a gallbladder. Opt for lean cuts of meat, poultry without skin, fish, and plant-based proteins instead.

3.   **Choose Healthy Fats:** Incorporate healthy fats from sources such as avocados, nuts, seeds, and olive oil. These fats are easier to digest and may help support bile production and fat absorption.

4.   **Focus on Fiber:** Include plenty of fiber-rich foods in your diet to promote regular bowel movements and prevent constipation. Choose fruits, vegetables, whole grains, legumes, and nuts to increase your fiber intake.

5.   **Small, Frequent Meals:** Eat smaller, more frequent meals throughout the day rather than large, heavy meals. This can help prevent overloading the digestive system and minimize symptoms such as bloating and discomfort.

6.   **Stay Hydrated:** Drink plenty of water throughout the day to help maintain hydration and support digestion. Aim for at least 8-10 cups of

fluid daily, and limit caffeine and alcohol, which can be dehydrating.

7.   **Monitor Symptoms:** Pay attention to how your body responds to different foods and adjust your diet accordingly. Keep a food journal to track symptoms and identify potential triggers that may exacerbate digestive issues.

8.   **Consider Digestive Enzymes:** Some women may benefit from taking digestive enzyme supplements with meals to aid in the digestion of fats and support overall digestive health.

9.   **Limit Gas-Producing Foods:** Reduce your intake of gas-producing foods such as beans, cabbage, broccoli, onions, and carbonated beverages, as they may contribute to bloating and discomfort.

A gallbladder post-surgical diet for women should focus on supporting digestion, minimizing discomfort, and promoting overall digestive health. By following these dietary guidelines and making gradual adjustments as needed, women can navigate life without a gallbladder with greater ease and comfort.

No Gallbladder Lifestyle For Women

Living without a gallbladder requires some adjustments to your lifestyle, particularly when it comes to diet and overall health management. Here are some key lifestyle tips for women adapting to life without a gallbladder:

1.   **Follow a Gallbladder-Friendly Diet:** Adopt a diet that is low in fat, particularly saturated and trans fats, to minimize digestive discomfort. Focus on lean proteins, healthy fats from sources like avocado and nuts, and high-fiber foods like fruits, vegetables, and whole grains. Avoiding large meals and spacing out meals throughout the day can also help manage symptoms.

2.   **Stay Hydrated:** Drink plenty of water throughout the day to support digestion and prevent dehydration. Aim for at least 8-10 cups of water

daily, and limit caffeinated and alcoholic beverages, which can contribute to dehydration.

3. **Gradually Reintroduce Foods:** After surgery, gradually reintroduce foods into your diet to gauge how your body responds. Keep a food diary to track any symptoms or reactions and identify potential trigger foods.

4. **Practice Portion Control:** Eating smaller, more frequent meals can help prevent digestive discomfort and promote better digestion. Focus on portion control and listen to your body's hunger and fullness cues.

5. **Be Mindful of Fat Intake:** While it's important to include some healthy fats in your diet, be mindful of your overall fat intake, as your body may have difficulty digesting large amounts of fat without a gallbladder. Opt for lean proteins, low-fat dairy products, and sources of healthy fats like olive oil and fatty fish.

6.   **Exercise Regularly:** Regular physical activity can support digestion, promote overall health, and help manage weight, which may be beneficial for women living without a gallbladder.

7.   **Manage Stress:** Stress can exacerbate digestive symptoms, so finding healthy ways to manage stress is essential. Practice relaxation techniques such as deep breathing, meditation, yoga, or tai chi to reduce stress and promote overall well-being.

8.   **Stay Informed:** Educate yourself about gallbladder health, post-surgical care, and dietary recommendations for individuals without a gallbladder. Stay in touch with your healthcare provider for regular check-ups and guidance on managing any ongoing symptoms or concerns.

9.   **Listen to Your Body:** Pay attention to how your body responds to different foods, activities,

and lifestyle choices. Trust your instincts and make adjustments as needed to support your overall health and well-being.

10.   **Seek Support:** Living without a gallbladder may present challenges, so don't hesitate to seek support from friends, family, or healthcare professionals. Joining support groups or online communities can also provide valuable encouragement and resources for managing life after gallbladder surgery.

By incorporating these lifestyle tips into your daily routine, women can effectively manage life without a gallbladder and enjoy improved digestive health and overall well-being. Remember to be patient with yourself as you navigate this transition and make adjustments to find what works best for you.

Foods to Avoid

After gallbladder removal surgery, it's advisable for women to avoid certain foods that may exacerbate digestive symptoms or discomfort. While individual tolerance may vary, here are some common foods to avoid in a gallbladder post-surgical diet:

1.   High-Fat Foods: Limit or avoid foods that are high in fat, as they can be difficult to digest without a gallbladder. This includes fried foods, fatty cuts of meat, full-fat dairy products, creamy sauces and dressings, and rich desserts.

2.   Spicy Foods: Spicy foods may irritate the digestive system and trigger symptoms such as heartburn, indigestion, or abdominal pain. Avoid foods seasoned with hot peppers, chili powder, garlic, or onions if they worsen symptoms.

3.　　Processed Foods: Processed foods, such as fast food, packaged snacks, and pre-packaged meals, often contain unhealthy fats, preservatives, and additives that can be hard on the digestive system. Whenever feasible, choose whole foods with little to no processing.

4.　　Highly Acidic Foods: Acidic foods and beverages may increase stomach acidity and exacerbate symptoms such as heartburn or acid reflux. Limit your intake of citrus fruits, tomatoes, vinegar, and acidic drinks like coffee, tea, and soda.

5.　　Carbonated Beverages: Carbonated beverages can contribute to bloating, gas, and abdominal discomfort. Avoid soda, sparkling water, and other fizzy drinks that may worsen digestive symptoms.

6.　　Raw Vegetables: Raw vegetables, particularly those that are high in fiber and difficult to digest, may cause bloating, gas, or cramping in some individuals. Steam or cook vegetables until they are soft and easily digestible.

7.   **Highly Processed Grains:** Highly processed grains, such as white bread, white rice, and refined pasta, lack fiber and nutrients and may contribute to digestive issues. Instead, go for whole grains like whole wheat bread, quinoa, and brown rice.

8.   **Alcohol and Caffeine:** Alcohol and caffeine can be irritating to the digestive tract and may stimulate bile production, leading to discomfort in some individuals. Limit your intake of alcoholic beverages, coffee, and caffeinated tea if they worsen symptoms.

9.   **High-Sugar Foods:** High-sugar foods and beverages, such as candy, pastries, sugary snacks, and sweetened drinks, can disrupt blood sugar levels and contribute to digestive discomfort.

Choose naturally sweetened alternatives like fresh fruit or small amounts of honey or maple syrup.

10.   Large Meals: Avoid consuming large meals, as they can overwhelm the digestive system and lead to discomfort. Instead, opt for smaller, more frequent meals throughout the day to support digestion and prevent symptoms.

By avoiding these foods and making dietary modifications as needed, women can better manage digestive symptoms and promote overall digestive health after gallbladder removal surgery. It's essential to listen to your body and adjust your diet based on individual tolerance and preferences.

Shopping List

1. Lean Proteins:

- Skinless chicken breast

- Turkey breast

- Fish (salmon, trout, tuna)

- Lean cuts of beef or pork (loin or sirloin)

- Eggs

- Tofu or tempeh

2. Fresh Produce:

- Leafy greens (spinach, kale, arugula)

- Cruciferous vegetables (broccoli, cauliflower, Brussels sprouts)

- Bell peppers (red, green, yellow)

- Zucchini

- Cucumbers

- Tomatoes

- Avocados

- Berries (strawberries, blueberries, raspberries)

- Apples

- Bananas

- Citrus fruits (lemons, oranges)

3. Whole Grains:

- Quinoa

- Brown rice

- Whole wheat pasta

- Rolled oats

- Whole grain bread or wraps

4. Healthy Fats:

- Olive oil

- Avocado oil

- Nuts (almonds, walnuts, pistachios)

- Seeds (like flaxseeds, pumpkin seeds, and chia seeds)

5. Dairy and Dairy Alternatives:

- Low-fat or fat-free yogurt

- Skim or low-fat milk

- Almond milk

- Soy milk

6. Beans and Legumes:

- Black beans
- Chickpeas
- Lentils
- Edamame

7. Herbs and Spices:

- Garlic
- Ginger
- Turmeric
- Basil
- Parsley
- Cilantro
- Cinnamon

8. Condiments and Flavorings:

- Balsamic vinegar
- Dijon mustard
- Low-sodium soy sauce
- Apple cider vinegar
- Maple syrup or honey

- Salsa (without added sugar)

9. Miscellaneous:

- Low-sodium broth or stock

- Herbal teas

- Dark chocolate (70% cocoa or higher, in moderation)

- Hummus

- Olives

10. Frozen Foods:

- Frozen fruits (berries, mango chunks, pineapple)

- Frozen vegetables (mixed vegetables, spinach, green beans)

11. Seafood:

- Shrimp

- Scallops

- Cod fillets

- Salmon or canned tuna (in water)

12. Sweeteners:

- Stevia

- Monk fruit sweetener

- Agave nectar (in moderation)

13. Grains and Legumes:

- Whole grain couscous

- Bulgur

- Farro

- Split peas

14. Dairy and Dairy Alternatives:

- Greek yogurt

- Cottage cheese

- Coconut milk (unsweetened)

15. Beverages:

- Sparkling water (plain or flavored, unsweetened)

- Herbal teas (peppermint, chamomile, ginger)

- Green tea

16. Snacks:

- Rice cakes

- Air-popped popcorn

- Veggie chips (made from kale, sweet potatoes or beets)

- Nut butter (almond, peanut, cashew)

17. Cooking Essentials:

- Cooking spray (such as avocado oil and olive oil)

- Low-sodium soy sauce or tamari

- Dried herbs and spices (oregano, thyme, paprika)

- Sea salt

- Black pepper

18. Gluten-Free Options:

- Gluten-free pasta (made from brown rice, quinoa, or chickpeas)

- Gluten-free bread or wraps

- Gluten-free oats

19. Healthy Snacks:

- Greek yogurt cups

- Raw veggies (like bell peppers, celery, or carrots) with hummus

- Cheese sticks or cheese slices (low-fat or reduced-fat)

- Nut and seed mix (the likes of walnuts, pumpkin seeds, almonds)

20. Miscellaneous:

- Nutritional yeast (for adding flavor and nutrients to dishes)

- Flaxseed meal (for adding omega-3 fatty acids and fiber to recipes)

- Vinegar (like balsamic vinegar or apple cider vinegar)

- Coconut oil

Remember to choose organic and fresh options whenever possible, and to read labels carefully to avoid added sugars, unhealthy fats, and artificial ingredients. With this shopping list, you'll be well-equipped to prepare delicious and gallbladder-friendly meals at home.

CHAPTER 2

Breakfast Recipes

1. Olive Oil and Sesame Asparagus

Ingredients:

- 1 bunch of asparagus, trimmed
- 1 tablespoon olive oil
- 1 tablespoon sesame seeds
- Salt and pepper to taste

Preparation:

1. Set the oven to 400°F (200°C) heat.

2. Place the trimmed asparagus spears on a baking sheet.

3. Drizzle with olive oil and sprinkle with sesame seeds, salt, and pepper.

4. Roast in the preheated oven for 10-12 minutes, or until the asparagus is tender.

Nutritional Value (per serving):

- Calories: 80

- Protein: 4g

- Fat: 6g

- Carbohydrates: 4g

- Fiber: 2g

Cooking Time: 10-12 minutes

Notes:

_____

_____

_____

_____

_____

_____

Progress Report:

_____

_____

_____

_____

_____

_____

2. Banana Cauliflower Smoothie

Ingredients:

- 1 ripe banana
- 1 cup steamed cauliflower florets
- ½ cup unsweetened almond milk
- 1 tablespoon almond butter
- 1 teaspoon of maple syrup or honey

Preparation:

1. Blend all the ingredients together.

2. Blend until smooth and creamy.

3. Add more almond milk if needed to reach desired consistency.

4. Pour the smoothie into a glass and serve cold.

Nutritional Value (per serving):

- Calories: 180
- Protein: 5g
- Fat: 8g
- Carbohydrates: 25g

- Fiber: 5g

Cooking Time: 5 minutes

Notes:

_____

_____

_____

_____

_____

_____

Progress Report:

_____

_____

_____

_____

_____

_____

3. Wholesome Buckwheat Pancakes

Ingredients:

- 1 cup buckwheat flour
- 1 teaspoon baking powder
- ¼ teaspoon salt
- 1 tablespoon honey or maple syrup
- 1 egg
- ¾ cup almond milk
- 1 tablespoon coconut oil, melted

Preparation:

1. In a large bowl, whisk together the buckwheat flour, baking powder, and salt.

2. In a separate bowl, whisk together the honey or maple syrup, egg, almond milk, and melted coconut oil.

3. After adding the wet components to the dry ingredients, mix just until incorporated.

4. Put a small amount of coconut oil on a nonstick skillet or griddle and heat it over medium heat.

5. Pour ¼ cup of batter onto the skillet for each pancake.

6. Cook until bubbles form on the surface, then flip and cook until golden brown on the other side.

Nutritional Value (per serving, 2 pancakes):

- Calories: 250
- Protein: 7g
- Fat: 8g
- Carbohydrates: 40g
- Fiber: 5g

Cooking Time: 15 minutes

Notes:

_____

_____

_____

_____

_____

_____

Progress Report:

_____

_____

_____

_____

_____

_____

4. Healthy Coconut Yogurt with Acai Berry Granola

Ingredients:

- 1 cup unsweetened coconut yogurt

- ¼ cup acai berry granola (store-bought or homemade)

- Fresh berries for topping (optional)

Preparation:

1. Spoon the coconut yogurt into a bowl.

2. Sprinkle the acai berry granola on top.

3. Add fresh berries for extra flavor and nutrition, if desired.

Nutritional Value (per serving):

- Calories: 200

- Protein: 5g

- Fat: 10g

- Carbohydrates: 20g

- Fiber: 5g

Cooking Time: 2 minutes

Notes:

_____

_____

_____

_____

_____

_____

Progress Report:

_____

_____

_____

_____

_____

_____

5. Healthy Hot Multigrains Bowl

Ingredients:

- ¼ cup cooked quinoa
- ¼ cup cooked steel-cut oats
- ¼ cup cooked amaranth
- ¼ cup unsweetened almond milk
- 1 tablespoon almond butter
- 1 tablespoon honey or maple syrup
- Fresh fruit for topping (such as sliced bananas or berries)

Preparation:

1. In a saucepan, combine the cooked quinoa, steel-cut oats, and amaranth.

2. Heat over medium heat until warmed through, stirring occasionally.

3. Stir in the almond milk, almond butter, and honey or maple syrup until well combined.

4. Transfer the multigrains mixture to a bowl and top with fresh fruit.

Nutritional Value (per serving):

- Calories: 300
- Protein: 8g
- Fat: 10g
- Carbohydrates: 45g
- Fiber: 7g

Cooking Time: 5 minutes

Notes:

_____

_____

_____

_____

_____

_____

Progress Report:

_____

_____

_____

_____

_____

_____

6. Pineapple Onion Omelet

Ingredients:

- 2 eggs
- ¼ cup diced pineapple
- ¼ cup diced onion
- 1 tablespoon olive oil
- Salt and pepper to taste

Preparation:

1. Beat the eggs thoroughly with a whisk in a bowl.

2. The olive oil should be heated in a non-stick skillet over medium heat.

3. Add diced pineapple and onion to the skillet and sauté for 2-3 minutes until softened.

4. Pour the beaten eggs over the pineapple and onion mixture in the skillet.

5. Cook until the edges are set, then carefully flip the omelet and cook for another 1-2 minutes until cooked through.

Nutritional Value (per serving):

- Calories: 200

- Protein: 12g

- Fat: 14g

- Carbohydrates: 10g

- Fiber: 2g

Cooking Time: 10 minutes

Notes:

_____

_____

_____

_____

_____

_____

Progress Report:

_____

_____

_____

_____

_____

_____

7. Blueberry Mint Fresh Toast

Ingredients:

- 2 slices whole grain bread
- ¼ cup fresh blueberries
- 1 tablespoon chopped fresh mint leaves
- 1 tablespoon honey or maple syrup
- Greek yogurt for topping (optional)

Preparation:

1. Toast the whole grain bread slices until golden brown.

2. In a small bowl, mix together the fresh blueberries, chopped mint leaves, and honey or maple syrup.

3. Spoon the blueberry mint mixture over the toasted bread slices.

4. Serve with a dollop of Greek yogurt on top, if desired.

Nutritional Value (per serving):

- Calories: 180
- Protein: 6g
- Fat: 2g
- Carbohydrates: 35g
- Fiber: 5g

Cooking Time: 5 minutes

Notes:

_____

_____

_____

_____

_____

_____

Progress Report:

_____

_____

_____

_____

_____

_____

8. Spiced Hummus Avocado Toast

Ingredients:

- 2 slices whole grain bread
- ½ ripe avocado, mashed
- 2 tablespoons hummus
- Pinch of paprika, cumin, and chili powder
- Salt and pepper to taste

Preparation:

1. Toast the whole grain bread slices until golden brown.

2. Spread mashed avocado evenly over each toast slice.

3. Spread hummus over the avocado layer.

4. Sprinkle with a pinch of paprika, cumin, and chili powder.

5. Season with salt and pepper to make it tasty.

Nutritional Value (per serving):

- Calories: 250
- Protein: 8g
- Fat: 12g
- Carbohydrates: 30g
- Fiber: 10g

Cooking Time: 5 minutes

Notes:

_____

_____

_____

_____

_____

_____

Progress Report:

_____

_____

_____

_____

_____

_____

9. Mango Ginger Smoothie

- 1 ripe mango, peeled and diced
- ½ inch fresh ginger, peeled and grated
- ½ cup unsweetened almond milk
- ½ cup plain Greek yogurt
- 1 tablespoon honey or maple syrup
- Ice cubes

Preparation:

1. In a blender, combine diced mango, grated ginger, almond milk, Greek yogurt, and honey or maple syrup.

2. Fill the blender with a few handfuls of ice cubes.

3. Blend until smooth and creamy.

4. Pour into a glass and serve immediately.

Nutritional Value (per serving):

- Calories: 200

- Protein: 10g

- Fat: 2g

- Carbohydrates: 40g

- Fiber: 5g

Cooking Time: 5 minutes

Notes:

_____

_____

_____

_____

_____

_____

Progress Report:

_____

_____

_____

_____

_____

_____

10. Kiwi Strawberry Banana Smoothie

Ingredients:

- 1 ripe banana
- 1 ripe kiwi, peeled and diced
- ½ cup fresh strawberries, hulled
- ½ cup unsweetened almond milk
- ½ cup plain Greek yogurt
- 1 tablespoon honey or maple syrup
- Ice cubes

Preparation:

1. In a blender, combine banana, kiwi, strawberries, almond milk, Greek yogurt, and honey or maple syrup.

2. Fill the blender with a few handfuls of ice cubes.

3. Blend until smooth and creamy.

4. Pour into a glass and serve immediately.

Nutritional Value (per serving):

- Calories: 180

- Protein: 8g

- Fat: 2g

- Carbohydrates: 35g

- Fiber: 5g

Cooking Time: 5 minutes

Notes:

_____

_____

_____

_____

_____

_____

Progress Report:

_____

_____

_____

_____

_____

_____

CHAPTER 3

Lunch Recipes

1. Garlic Turkey Breast with Lemon

Ingredients:

- 2 turkey breast fillets

- 2 cloves garlic, minced

- 1 tablespoon olive oil

- Juice of 1 lemon

- Salt and pepper to taste

Preparation:

1. Preheat the oven to 375°F (190°C).

2. In a small bowl, mix minced garlic, olive oil, lemon juice, salt, and pepper.

3. Place turkey breast fillets in a baking dish and pour the garlic-lemon mixture over them.

4. Bake for 25-30 minutes or until turkey is cooked through.

Nutritional Value (per serving):
- Calories: 200
- Protein: 25g
- Fat: 8g
- Carbohydrates: 2g
- Fiber: 0g

Cooking Time: 30 minutes

Notes:

_____

_____

_____

_____

_____

_____

Progress Report:

_____

_____

_____

_____

_____

_____

2. Sautéed Turkey with Cabbage

Ingredients:

- 1 lb turkey breast, thinly sliced
- 2 cups shredded cabbage
- 2 cloves garlic, minced
- 1 tablespoon olive oil
- Salt and pepper to taste

Preparation:

1. The olive oil should be heated in a large skillet over medium heat.

2. Add minced garlic and cook until fragrant.

3. Add thinly sliced turkey breast to the skillet and cook until browned and cooked through.

4. Add shredded cabbage to the skillet and sauté until wilted.

5. Season with salt and pepper to make it tasty.

Nutritional Value (per serving):

- Calories: 250

- Protein: 30g

- Fat: 10g

- Carbohydrates: 8g

- Fiber: 4g

Cooking Time: 15 minutes

Notes:

_____

_____

_____

_____

_____

_____

Progress Report:

_____

_____

_____

_____

_____

_____

3. Baked Lemon Salmon with Zucchini

Ingredients:

- 2 salmon fillets

- 2 medium zucchinis, sliced

- 1 lemon, thinly sliced

- 2 tablespoons olive oil

- Salt and pepper to taste

Preparation:

1. Preheat the oven to 375°F (190°C).

2. On a baking sheet covered with parchment paper, arrange the salmon fillets.

3. Arrange sliced zucchini and lemon slices around the salmon.

4. Drizzle olive oil over salmon, zucchini, and lemon slices. Season with salt and pepper.

5. Bake for 15-20 minutes or until salmon is cooked through and zucchini is tender.

Nutritional Value (per serving):

- Calories: 300

- Protein: 25g

- Fat: 18g

- Carbohydrates: 10g

- Fiber: 4g

Cooking Time: 20 minutes

Notes:

_____

_____

_____

_____

_____

_____

Progress Report:

_____

_____

_____

_____

_____

_____

4. Kale and Cottage Pasta

Ingredients:

- 8 oz whole wheat pasta
- 2 cups chopped kale
- 1 cup low-fat cottage cheese
- 2 cloves garlic, minced
- 1 tablespoon olive oil
- Salt and pepper to taste

Preparation:

1. Cook pasta as directed on the package until it's al dente. Drain and set aside.

2. A skillet with medium heat should be used to heat the olive oil. After adding, sauté the minced garlic until fragrant.

3. Add chopped kale to the skillet and sauté until wilted.

4. Stir in cooked pasta and cottage cheese until heated through.

5. Season with salt and pepper to make it tasty.

Nutritional Value (per serving):

- Calories: 350

- Protein: 20g

- Fat: 8g

- Carbohydrates: 50g

- Fiber: 8g

Cooking Time: 20 minutes

Notes:

_____

_____

_____

_____

_____

_____

Progress Report:

_____

_____

_____

_____

_____

_____

5. Pork Loins with Leeks

Ingredients:

- 4 pork loin chops
- 2 leeks, thinly sliced
- 2 tablespoons olive oil
- 2 cloves garlic, minced
- Salt and pepper to taste

Preparation:

1. Season pork loin chops with salt and pepper.

2. A skillet with medium heat should be used to heat the olive oil. Sauté the minced garlic until fragrant.

3. Add pork loin chops to the skillet and cook for 4-5 minutes on each side until browned and cooked through.

4. Add sliced leeks to the skillet and sauté until tender.

5. Serve pork loin chops with sautéed leeks.

Nutritional Value (per serving):

- Calories: 300

- Protein: 30g

- Fat: 15g

- Carbohydrates: 10g

- Fiber: 2g

Cooking Time: 20 minutes

Notes:

_____

_____

_____

_____

_____

_____

Progress Report:

_____

_____

_____

_____

_____

_____

6. Beef and Sweet Potato Enchilada Casserole

Ingredients:

- 1 lb lean ground beef
- 2 chopped and peeled sweet potatoes
- 1 onion, diced
- 2 cloves garlic, minced
- 1 can (15 oz) of drained and rinsed black beans
- 1 can (15 oz) enchilada sauce
- 1 cup shredded cheddar cheese
- Salt and pepper to taste

Preparation:

1. Preheat the oven to 375°F (190°C). Grease a baking dish.

2. The ground beef should be cooked in a large skillet over medium heat. Drain excess fat.

3. Add diced sweet potatoes, diced onion, and minced garlic to the skillet. Cook until vegetables are tender.

4. Stir in black beans and enchilada sauce until well combined.

5. Transfer the beef and sweet potato mixture to the prepared baking dish. Top with shredded cheddar cheese.

6. Bake the cheese for 25 to 30 minutes, or until it is bubbling and melted..

Nutritional Value (per serving):

- Calories: 400

- Protein: 25g

- Fat: 15g

- Carbohydrates: 40g

- Fiber: 8g

Cooking Time: 40 minutes

Notes:

_____

_____

_____

_____

_____

_____

Progress Report:

_____

_____

_____

_____

_____

_____

7. Green Pesto Pasta

Ingredients:

- 8 oz whole wheat pasta
- 1 cup fresh basil leaves
- ¼ cup pine nuts
- 2 cloves garlic
- ¼ cup grated Parmesan cheese
- ¼ cup olive oil
- Salt and pepper to taste

Preparation:

1. Pasta should be cooked as directed on the package until it is al dente. Drain and set aside.

2. In a food processor, combine basil leaves, pine nuts, garlic, Parmesan cheese, olive oil, salt, and pepper. Blend until smooth.

3. Toss cooked pasta with pesto sauce until well coated.

4. Serve hot or cold.

Nutritional Value (per serving):

- Calories: 350

- Protein: 10g

- Fat: 20g

- Carbohydrates: 30g

- Fiber: 5g

Cooking Time: 20 minutes

8. Rice and Chicken Soup

Ingredients:

- 1 cup cooked brown rice

- 1 cup of cooked chicken breast, shredded

- 2 carrots, diced

- 2 celery stalks, diced

- 1 onion, diced

- 2 cloves garlic, minced

- 6 cups low-sodium chicken broth

- 1 bay leaf

- Salt and pepper to taste

Preparation:

1. Pour olive oil into a big pot and warm it up to medium. Incorporate chopped garlic, diced onion, carrots, and celery. Cook until vegetables are softened.

2. Add shredded chicken breast, cooked brown rice, chicken broth, and bay leaf to the pot. Bring to a boil.

3. Reduce heat and simmer for 20-25 minutes until flavors are blended.

4. Season with salt and pepper to taste before serving.

Nutritional Value (per serving):
- Calories: 250
- Protein: 20g
- Fat: 5g
- Carbohydrates: 30g
- Fiber: 5g

Cooking Time: 30 minutes

Notes:

_____

_____

_____

_____

_____

_____

Progress Report:

_____

_____

_____

_____

_____

_____

9. Fresh Kale Garlic Soup

Ingredients:

- 4 cups chopped kale
- 1 onion, diced
- 2 cloves garlic, minced
- 4 cups low-sodium vegetable broth
- 1 tablespoon olive oil
- Salt and pepper to taste

Preparation:

1. In a large pot, heat olive oil over medium heat. Add diced onion and minced garlic. Cook until fragrant.

2. Add chopped kale to the pot and sauté until wilted.

3. Pour vegetable broth into the pot and bring to a boil.

4. Reduce heat and simmer for 15-20 minutes until kale is tender.

5. Season with salt and pepper to taste before serving.

Nutritional Value (per serving):
- Calories: 150
- Protein: 5g
- Fat: 5g
- Carbohydrates: 20g
- Fiber: 5g

Cooking Time: 25 minutes

Notes:

_____

_____

_____

_____

_____

_____

Progress Report:

_____

_____

_____

_____

_____

_____

10. Spinach Soup

Ingredients:

- 4 cups fresh spinach leaves
- 1 onion, diced
- 2 cloves garlic, minced
- 4 cups low-sodium vegetable broth
- 1 tablespoon olive oil
- Salt and pepper to taste

Preparation:

1. Warm up the olive oil in a big pot over medium heat. Add diced onion and minced garlic. Cook until fragrant.

2. Add fresh spinach leaves to the pot and sauté until wilted.

3. Fill the saucepan with veggie broth and heat it until it boils.

4. Reduce heat and simmer for 10-15 minutes until spinach is tender.

5. Before serving, season to taste with salt and pepper.

Nutritional Value (per serving):
- Calories: 100
- Protein: 5g
- Fat: 5g
- Carbohydrates: 15g
- Fiber: 5g

Cooking Time: 20 minutes

Notes:

_____

_____

_____

_____

_____

_____

Progress Report:

_____

_____

_____

_____

_____

_____

CHAPTER 4

Dinner Recipes

1. Thai Tofu Broth

Ingredients:

- 1 block of cubed (14 oz) firm tofu
- 4 cups vegetable broth
- 1 can (14 oz) coconut milk
- Thai red curry paste (2 tablespoons)
- 1 tablespoon soy sauce
- 1 tablespoon fresh lime juice
- 1 tablespoon fresh cilantro, chopped
- Salt and pepper to taste

Preparation:

1. In a large pot, combine vegetable broth, coconut milk, and Thai red curry paste. Bring to a simmer.

2. Add cubed tofu to the broth mixture and cook for 10 minutes.

3. Stir in soy sauce, lime juice, chopped cilantro, salt, and pepper.

4. Serve hot and enjoy.

Nutritional Value (per serving):

- Calories: 250
- Protein: 15g
- Fat: 18g
- Carbohydrates: 10g
- Fiber: 2g

Cooking Time: 15 minutes

Notes:

_____

_____

_____

_____

_____

_____

Progress Report:

_____

_____

_____

_____

_____

_____

2. Salad with Strawberries and Goat Cheese

Ingredients:

- 4 cups mixed salad greens
- 1 cup sliced strawberries
- ¼ cup crumbled goat cheese
- 2 tablespoons balsamic vinaigrette

Preparation:

1. In a large bowl, combine mixed salad greens, sliced strawberries, and crumbled goat cheese.

2. Drizzle with balsamic vinaigrette and toss to coat evenly.

3. Serve immediately.

Nutritional Value (per serving):

- Calories: 150
- Protein: 5g
- Fat: 8g
- Carbohydrates: 15g

- Fiber: 4g

Cooking Time: 5 minutes

Notes:

_____

_____

_____

_____

_____

_____

Progress Report:

_____

_____

_____

_____

_____

_____

3. Cantaloupe Salad

- 2 cups cubed cantaloupe
- 1 cup diced cucumber
- ¼ cup finely chopped, fresh mint leaves
- 1 tablespoon lime juice
- 1 tablespoon honey
- Pinch of salt

Preparation:

1. In a large bowl, combine cubed cantaloupe, diced cucumber, and chopped fresh mint leaves.

2. In a small bowl, whisk together lime juice, honey, and a pinch of salt.

3. Pour the dressing over the salad and toss to coat evenly.

4. Serve chilled.

Nutritional Value (per serving):

- Calories: 100

- Protein: 1g

- Fat: 0g

- Carbohydrates: 25g

- Fiber: 2g

Cooking Time: 10 minutes

Notes:

_____

_____

_____

_____

_____

_____

Progress Report:

_____

_____

_____

_____

_____

_____

4. Lentil Super Salad

Ingredients:

- 1 cup cooked lentils
- ½ cup diced bell pepper
- ½ cup diced cucumber
- ¼ cup chopped red onion
- ¼ cup chopped fresh parsley
- 2 tablespoons olive oil
- 1 tablespoon lemon juice
- Salt and pepper to taste

Preparation:

1. In a large bowl, combine cooked lentils, diced bell pepper, diced cucumber, chopped red onion, and chopped fresh parsley.

2. Mix the lemon juice, olive oil, salt, and pepper in a small bowl.

3. Pour the dressing over the salad and toss to coat evenly.

4. It can be served cold or warm.

Nutritional Value (per serving):

- Calories: 200
- Protein: 10g
- Fat: 8g
- Carbohydrates: 25g
- Fiber: 8g

Cooking Time: 15 minutes

Notes:

_____

_____

_____

_____

_____

_____

Progress Report:

_____

_____

_____

_____

_____

_____

5. Broccoli with Garlic Sauce

Ingredients:

- 4 cups broccoli florets

- 2 cloves garlic, minced

- 2 tablespoons soy sauce

- 1 tablespoon rice vinegar

- 1 tablespoon honey or maple syrup

- 1 tablespoon sesame oil

- Sesame seeds for garnish

Preparation:

1. Steam broccoli florets until tender-crisp, about 5 minutes. Drain and set aside.

2. In a small bowl, whisk together minced garlic, soy sauce, rice vinegar, honey or maple syrup, and sesame oil.

3. Heat a skillet over medium heat and add the sauce mixture. Cook for 1-2 minutes until fragrant.

4. Add steamed broccoli to the skillet and toss to coat evenly with the sauce.

5. Before serving, sprinkle with sesame seeds.

Nutritional Value (per serving):

- Calories: 100

- Protein: 5g

- Fat: 4g

- Carbohydrates: 15g

- Fiber: 5g

Cooking Time: 10 minutes

Notes:

_____

_____

_____

_____

_____

_____

Progress Report:

_____

_____

_____

_____

_____

_____

6. Sautéed Green Beans

Ingredients:

- 2 cups green beans, trimmed
- 2 cloves garlic, minced
- 1 tablespoon olive oil
- Salt and pepper to taste

Preparation:

1. A skillet with medium heat should be used to heat the olive oil. Add the chopped garlic and cook it for one minute.

2. Add green beans to the skillet and sauté for 5-7 minutes, or until tender-crisp.

3. Season with salt and pepper to make it tasty.

4. Serve hot.

Nutritional Value (per serving):

- Calories: 50
- Protein: 2g
- Fat: 3g

- Carbohydrates: 7g

- Fiber: 3g

Cooking Time: 10 minutes

Notes:

_____

_____

_____

_____

_____

_____

Progress Report:

_____

_____

_____

_____

_____

_____

7. Coconut and Pecan Sweet Potatoes

Ingredients:

- 2 large sweet potatoes, peeled and cubed
- ¼ cup shredded coconut
- ¼ cup chopped pecans
- 2 tablespoons maple syrup
- 1 tablespoon coconut oil, melted
- 1 teaspoon cinnamon
- Pinch of salt

Preparation:

1. Preheat the oven to 400°F (200°C). Put parchment paper on one side of a baking sheet.

2. In a large bowl, toss sweet potato cubes with shredded coconut, chopped pecans, maple syrup, melted coconut oil, cinnamon, and a pinch of salt until evenly coated.

3. Spread the sweet potato mixture in a single layer on the prepared baking sheet.

4. Stir the sweet potatoes halfway during the baking time of 25 to 30 minutes, or until they are soft and caramelized.

5. Serve hot.

Nutritional Value (per serving):

- Calories: 200

- Protein: 3g

- Fat: 9g

- Carbohydrates: 30g

- Fiber: 5g

Cooking Time: 30 minutes

Notes:

_____

_____

_____

_____

_____

Progress Report:

_____

_____

_____

_____

_____

8. Parsley Root Veg Stew

Ingredients:

- 2 cups diced parsley root
- 1 cup diced carrots
- 1 cup diced potatoes
- 1 cup diced onions
- 4 cups vegetable broth
- 2 cloves garlic, minced
- 2 tablespoons olive oil
- 1 teaspoon dried thyme
- Salt and pepper to taste

Preparation:

1. Over medium heat, warm up the olive oil in a big pot. Add minced garlic and diced onions, and sauté until onions are translucent.

2. Add diced parsley root, carrots, and potatoes to the pot, and cook for 5 minutes, stirring occasionally.

3. Pour vegetable broth into the pot, and add dried thyme, salt, and pepper.

4. Vegetables should be soft after 20 to 25 minutes of simmering the stew after bringing it to a boil.

5. Serve hot and enjoy.

Nutritional Value (per serving):

- Calories: 180
- Protein: 4g
- Fat: 5g
- Carbohydrates: 30g
- Fiber: 6g

Cooking Time: 35 minutes

Notes:

_____

_____

_____

_____

_____

_____

Progress Report:

_____

_____

_____

_____

_____

_____

9. Chickpea Salad Wrap

Ingredients:

- 1 can (15 oz) chickpeas, drained and rinsed
- ½ cup diced cucumber
- ½ cup diced tomatoes
- ¼ cup diced red onion
- 2 tablespoons chopped fresh parsley
- 2 tablespoons olive oil
- 1 tablespoon lemon juice
- 1 teaspoon ground cumin
- Salt and pepper to taste
- 4 whole wheat tortillas

Preparation:

1. In a large bowl, combine chickpeas, diced cucumber, diced tomatoes, diced red onion, and chopped fresh parsley.

2. In a small bowl, whisk together olive oil, lemon juice, ground cumin, salt, and pepper.

3. Pour the dressing over the chickpea mixture and toss to coat evenly.

4. Divide the chickpea salad among the whole wheat tortillas, and wrap them up.

5. Serve immediately or wrap in foil for later.

Nutritional Value (per serving):

- Calories: 250
- Protein: 8g
- Fat: 10g
- Carbohydrates: 35g
- Fiber: 8g

Cooking Time: 15 minutes

Notes:

_____

_____

_____

_____

_____

_____

Progress Report:

_____

_____

_____

_____

_____

_____

10. Rotisserie Chicken Noodle Soup

Ingredients:

- 1 rotisserie chicken, shredded
- 6 cups low-sodium chicken broth
- 2 carrots, sliced
- 2 celery stalks, sliced
- 1 onion, diced
- 2 cloves garlic, minced
- 2 cups cooked egg noodles
- 2 tablespoons chopped fresh parsley
- Salt and pepper to taste

Preparation:

1. In a large pot, combine shredded rotisserie chicken, low-sodium chicken broth, sliced carrots, sliced celery, diced onion, and minced garlic.

2. Bring the soup to a boil, then reduce heat and simmer for 15-20 minutes, or until vegetables are tender.

3. Add cooked egg noodles to the pot, and simmer for an additional 5 minutes.

4. Season the soup with chopped fresh parsley, salt, and pepper before serving.

5. Serve hot and enjoy.

Nutritional Value (per serving):

- Calories: 300
- Protein: 20g
- Fat: 10g
- Carbohydrates: 25g
- Fiber: 3g

Cooking Time: 30 minutes

Notes:

_____

_____

_____

_____

_____

_____

Progress Report:

_____

_____

_____

_____

_____

_____

CHAPTER 5

Snack Recipes

1. Buffalo Chicken Dip

Ingredients:

- 2 cups shredded cooked chicken breast

- ½ cup hot sauce

- ¼ cup Greek yogurt

- ¼ cup cream cheese, softened

- ¼ cup shredded cheddar cheese

- ¼ cup chopped green onions

- 1 teaspoon garlic powder

- 1 teaspoon onion powder

- Salt and pepper to taste

Preparation:

1. Set the oven to 350°F (175°C) heat.

2. In a mixing bowl, combine shredded chicken, hot sauce, Greek yogurt, cream cheese, shredded

cheddar cheese, chopped green onions, garlic powder, onion powder, salt, and pepper.

3. Evenly spread out the ingredients after transferring it to a baking dish.

4. Bake for 20-25 minutes, or until the dip is bubbly and lightly browned on top.

5. Serve hot with carrot sticks or celery.

Nutritional Value (per serving):

- Calories: 150

- Protein: 15g

- Fat: 8g

- Carbohydrates: 4g

- Fiber: 1g

Cooking Time: 25 minutes

Notes:

_____

_____

_____

_____

_____

_____

Progress Report:

_____

_____

_____

_____

_____

_____

2. Savory Collard Chips

Ingredients:

- 6 large collard green leaves

- 1 tablespoon olive oil

- Salt and pepper to taste

Preparation:

1. Set the oven to 350°F (175°C) heat.

2. Remove the stems from the collard green leaves and tear them into chip-sized pieces.

3. Place the collard green pieces on a baking sheet lined with parchment paper.

4. Drizzle olive oil over the collard green pieces and sprinkle with salt and pepper.

5. Bake for 10-12 minutes, or until the collard chips are crispy.

6. Let them cool before serving.

Nutritional Value (per serving):

- Calories: 50
- Protein: 3g
- Fat: 3g
- Carbohydrates: 5g
- Fiber: 3g

Cooking Time: 12 minutes

Notes:

_____

_____

_____

_____

_____

_____

Progress Report:

_____

_____

_____

_____

_____

_____

3. Spiced Apple Crisps

Ingredients:

- 2 apples, thinly sliced
- 1 tablespoon lemon juice
- 1 teaspoon ground cinnamon
- ½ teaspoon ground nutmeg
- ¼ teaspoon ground cloves

Preparation:

1. Preheat the oven to 200°F (95°C).

2. In a bowl, toss the thinly sliced apples with lemon juice, ground cinnamon, ground nutmeg, and ground cloves until evenly coated.

3. Place the apple slices on a baking sheet lined with parchment paper, making sure they are not overlapping.

4. Bake for 2-3 hours, or until the apple slices are dried and crispy.

5. Let them cool completely before serving.

Nutritional Value (per serving):

- Calories: 50

- Protein: 0g

- Fat: 0g

- Carbohydrates: 15g

- Fiber: 3g

Cooking Time: 2-3 hours

Notes:

_____

_____

_____

_____

_____

_____

Progress Report:

_____

_____

_____

_____

_____

_____

4. Avocado and Pea Dip with Carrots

Ingredients:

- 1 ripe avocado, peeled and pitted
- 1 cup frozen peas, thawed
- 1 tablespoon lemon juice
- 1 clove garlic, minced
- 2 tablespoons chopped fresh cilantro
- Salt and pepper to taste
- Carrot sticks for serving

Preparation:

1. In a food processor, combine the ripe avocado, thawed peas, lemon juice, minced garlic, chopped fresh cilantro, salt, and pepper.

2. Process until smooth and creamy.

3. Transfer the dip to a serving bowl and serve with carrot sticks.

Nutritional Value (per serving):

- Calories: 80

- Protein: 2g

- Fat: 5g

- Carbohydrates: 8g

- Fiber: 4g

Cooking Time: 10 minutes

Notes:

_____

_____

_____

_____

_____

_____

Progress Report:

_____

_____

_____

_____

_____

_____

5. Roasted Sweet Potato

Ingredients:

- 2 medium sweet potatoes, peeled and cubed
- 1 tablespoon olive oil
- 1 teaspoon smoked paprika
- ½ teaspoon garlic powder
- ½ teaspoon onion powder
- Salt and pepper to taste

Preparation:

1. Set the oven to 400°F (200°C) heat.

2. In a bowl, toss the cubed sweet potatoes with olive oil, smoked paprika, garlic powder, onion powder, salt, and pepper until evenly coated.

3. Spread the sweet potato cubes in a single layer on a baking sheet lined with parchment paper.

4. Roast the sweet potatoes for 25 to 30 minutes, stirring halfway through, or until they are soft and caramelized.

5. You can serve it hot or cold.

Nutritional Value (per serving):

- Calories: 100
- Protein: 1g
- Fat: 4g
- Carbohydrates: 17g
- Fiber: 3g

Cooking Time: 30 minutes

Notes:

_____

_____

_____

_____

_____

_____

Progress Report:

_____

_____

_____

_____

_____

_____

6. Spiced and Creamed Corn Snack

Ingredients:

- 2 cups frozen corn kernels, thawed
- ¼ cup coconut cream
- 1 teaspoon chili powder
- ½ teaspoon ground cumin
- ½ teaspoon smoked paprika
- Salt and pepper to taste

Preparation:

1. In a skillet over medium heat, add the thawed corn kernels and cook until slightly golden brown, about 5-7 minutes.

2. Stir in coconut cream, chili powder, ground cumin, smoked paprika, salt, and pepper.

3. Cook for an additional 2-3 minutes, or until the corn is coated with the cream mixture and heated through.

4. Before serving, remove from the heat and allow to cool slightly.

Nutritional Value (per serving):
  - Calories: 120
  - Protein: 2g
  - Fat: 5g
  - Carbohydrates: 20g
  - Fiber: 3g

Cooking Time: 10 minutes

Notes:

_____

_____

_____

_____

_____

_____

Progress Report:

_____

_____

_____

_____

_____

_____

7. Grain-Free Mixed Seed Crackers

Ingredients:

- 1 cup almond flour
- ¼ cup ground flaxseeds
- ¼ cup chia seeds
- ¼ cup sesame seeds
- ¼ cup sunflower seeds
- ¼ cup pumpkin seeds
- ½ teaspoon garlic powder
- ½ teaspoon onion powder
- ¼ teaspoon sea salt
- 2 tablespoons olive oil
- ¼ cup water

Preparation:

1. Preheat the oven to 325°F (160°C) and line a baking sheet with parchment paper.

2. In a large bowl, combine almond flour, ground flaxseeds, chia seeds, sesame seeds, sunflower

seeds, pumpkin seeds, garlic powder, onion powder, and sea salt.

3. Add olive oil and water to the bowl and mix until a dough forms.

4. Place the dough between two sheets of parchment paper and roll it out into a thin rectangle.

5. Using a pizza cutter, cut the dough into small squares to form crackers.

6. Transfer the crackers to the prepared baking sheet and bake for 15-20 minutes, or until golden brown and crispy.

7. Let them cool completely before serving.

Nutritional Value (per serving):
- Calories: 100
- Protein: 4g
- Fat: 8g
- Carbohydrates: 5g
- Fiber: 3g

Cooking Time: 20 minutes

Notes:

_____

_____

_____

_____

_____

_____

Progress Report:

_____

_____

_____

_____

_____

_____

8. Taro Chips

Ingredients:

- 2 medium taro roots, peeled and thinly sliced
- 2 tablespoons olive oil
- Salt to taste

Preparation:

1. Set the oven to 375°F (190°C) heat and put parchment paper on one side of a baking sheet.

2. In a bowl, toss the thinly sliced taro roots with olive oil until evenly coated.

3. After the baking sheet is ready, arrange the taro slices in a single layer.

4. Sprinkle with salt.

5. Bake for 20-25 minutes, or until the taro chips are golden brown and crispy.

6. Let them cool before serving.

Nutritional Value (per serving):

- Calories: 80

- Protein: 1g

- Fat: 4g

- Carbohydrates: 10g

- Fiber: 2g

Cooking Time: 25 minutes

Notes:

_____

_____

_____

_____

_____

_____

Progress Report:

_____

_____

_____

_____

_____

_____

9. Spiced Mango Trail Mix

Ingredients:

- 1 cup of dried and sliced mango slices
- ½ cup raw almonds
- ½ cup raw cashews
- ¼ cup pumpkin seeds
- ¼ cup sunflower seeds
- 1 teaspoon ground cinnamon
- ½ teaspoon ground ginger
- ¼ teaspoon ground nutmeg
- Pinch of salt

Preparation:

1. In a large bowl, combine chopped dried mango slices, raw almonds, raw cashews, pumpkin seeds, sunflower seeds, ground cinnamon, ground ginger, ground nutmeg, and a pinch of salt.

2. Toss until all ingredients are well mixed.

3. Divide the trail mix into individual servings or store in an airtight container.

Nutritional Value (per serving):

- Calories: 150

- Protein: 5g

- Fat: 10g

- Carbohydrates: 15g

- Fiber: 3g

Cooking Time: None

Notes:

_____

_____

_____

_____

_____

_____

Progress Report:

_____

_____

_____

_____

_____

_____

10. Thai Style Eggplant Dip

Ingredients:

- 2 large eggplants

- 2 cloves garlic, minced

- 1 tablespoon olive oil

- 2 tablespoons tahini

- 1 tablespoon lemon juice

- 1 teaspoon soy sauce

- ½ teaspoon ground cumin

- Salt and pepper to taste

- Chopped fresh cilantro for garnish

Preparation:

1. Set the oven to 400°F (200°C) heat.

2. Cut the eggplants in half lengthwise, then use a knife to score the flesh.

3. With the cut side facing up, place the eggplant halves on a baking sheet covered with parchment paper.

4. In a small bowl, mix minced garlic, olive oil, tahini, lemon juice, soy sauce, ground cumin, salt, and pepper.

5. Brush the mixture over the scored flesh of the eggplants.

6. Bake for 30-40 minutes, or until the eggplants are tender and golden brown.

7. Take them out of the oven and give them some time to cool.

8. Scoop out the flesh of the eggplants and transfer to a food processor.

9. Blend until smooth and creamy.

10. Garnish with chopped fresh cilantro before serving.

Nutritional Value (per serving):
- Calories: 100
- Protein: 2g
- Fat: 6g
- Carbohydrates: 10g
- Fiber: 5g

Cooking Time: 40 minutes

Notes:

_____

_____

_____

_____

_____

_____

Progress Report:

_____

_____

_____

_____

_____

30 Day Meal Plan

Week 1

Day 1:

Breakfast: Wholesome Buckwheat Pancakes

Lunch: Garlic Turkey Breast with Lemon

Dinner: Thai Tofu Broth

Snack: Buffalo Chicken Dip

Day 2:

Breakfast: Banana Cauliflower Smoothie

Lunch: Baked Lemon Salmon with Zucchini

Dinner: Salad with Strawberries and Goat Cheese

Snack: Savory Collard Chips

Day 3:

Breakfast: Healthy Coconut Yogurt with Acai Berry Granola

Lunch: Kale and Cottage Pasta

Dinner: Cantaloupe Salad

Snack: Spiced Apple Crisps

Day 4:

Breakfast: Kiwi Strawberry Banana Smoothie

Lunch: Beef and Sweet Potato Enchilada Casserole

Dinner: Lentil Super Salad

Snack: Avocado and Pea Dip with Carrots

Day 5:

Breakfast: Mango Ginger Smoothie

Lunch: Green Pesto Pasta

Dinner: Broccoli with Garlic Sauce

Snack: Roasted Sweet Potato

Day 6:

Breakfast: Olive Oil and Sesame Asparagus

Lunch: Rice and Chicken Soup

Dinner: Sautéed Green Beans

Snack: Spiced and Creamed Corn Snack

Day 7:

Breakfast: Pineapple Onion Omelet

Lunch: Fresh Kale Garlic Soup

Dinner: Coconut and Pecan Sweet Potatoes

Snack: Grain-Free Mixed Seed Crackers

Week 2

Breakfast: Blueberry Mint Fresh Toast

Lunch: Spinach Soup

Dinner: Parsley Root Veg Stew

Snack: Taro Chips

Breakfast: Spiced Hummus Avocado Toast

Lunch: Pork Loins with Leeks

Dinner: Chickpea Salad Wrap

Snack: Spiced Mango Trail Mix

Breakfast: Healthy Hot Multigrains Bowl

Lunch: Green Pesto Pasta

Dinner: Rotisserie Chicken Noodle Soup

Snack: Thai Style Eggplant Dip

Day 11:

Breakfast: Olive Oil and Sesame Asparagus

Lunch: Rice and Chicken Soup

Dinner: Sautéed Green Beans

Snack: Spiced and Creamed Corn Snack

Day 12:

Breakfast: Pineapple Onion Omelet

Lunch: Fresh Kale Garlic Soup

Dinner: Coconut and Pecan Sweet Potatoes

Snack: Grain-Free Mixed Seed Crackers

Day 13:

Breakfast: Blueberry Mint Fresh Toast

Lunch: Spinach Soup

Dinner: Parsley Root Veg Stew

Snack: Taro Chips

Day 14:

Breakfast: Spiced Hummus Avocado Toast

Lunch: Pork Loins with Leeks

Dinner: Chickpea Salad Wrap

Snack: Spiced Mango Trail Mix

Week 3

Breakfast: Healthy Hot Multigrains Bowl

Lunch: Green Pesto Pasta

Dinner: Rotisserie Chicken Noodle Soup

Snack: Thai Style Eggplant Dip

Breakfast: Wholesome Buckwheat Pancakes

Lunch: Garlic Turkey Breast with Lemon

Dinner: Thai Tofu Broth

Snack: Buffalo Chicken Dip

Breakfast: Banana Cauliflower Smoothie

Lunch: Baked Lemon Salmon with Zucchini

Dinner: Salad with Strawberries and Goat Cheese

Snack: Savory Collard Chips

Day 18:

Breakfast: Healthy Coconut Yogurt with Acai Berry Granola

Lunch: Kale and Cottage Pasta

Dinner: Cantaloupe Salad

Snack: Spiced Apple Crisps

Day 19:

Breakfast: Kiwi Strawberry Banana Smoothie

Lunch: Beef and Sweet Potato Enchilada Casserole

Dinner: Lentil Super Salad

Snack: Avocado and Pea Dip with Carrots

Day 20:

Breakfast: Mango Ginger Smoothie

Lunch: Green Pesto Pasta

Dinner: Broccoli with Garlic Sauce

Snack: Roasted Sweet Potato

Day 21:

Breakfast: Wholesome Buckwheat Pancakes

Lunch: Garlic Turkey Breast with Lemon

Dinner: Thai Tofu Broth

Snack: Buffalo Chicken Dip

Week 4

Breakfast: Banana Cauliflower Smoothie

Lunch: Baked Lemon Salmon with Zucchini

Dinner: Salad with Strawberries and Goat Cheese

Snack: Savory Collard Chips

Breakfast: Healthy Coconut Yogurt with Acai Berry Granola

Lunch: Kale and Cottage Pasta

Dinner: Cantaloupe Salad

Snack: Spiced Apple Crisps

Breakfast: Kiwi Strawberry Banana Smoothie

Lunch: Beef and Sweet Potato Enchilada Casserole

Dinner: Lentil Super Salad

Snack: Avocado and Pea Dip with Carrots

Day 25:

Breakfast: Mango Ginger Smoothie

Lunch: Green Pesto Pasta

Dinner: Broccoli with Garlic Sauce

Snack: Roasted Sweet Potato

Day 26:

Breakfast: Olive Oil and Sesame Asparagus

Lunch: Rice and Chicken Soup

Dinner: Sautéed Green Beans

Snack: Spiced and Creamed Corn Snack

Day 27:

Breakfast: Pineapple Onion Omelet

Lunch: Fresh Kale Garlic Soup

Dinner: Coconut and Pecan Sweet Potatoes

Snack: Grain-Free Mixed Seed Crackers

Day 28:

Breakfast: Blueberry Mint Fresh Toast

Lunch: Spinach Soup

Dinner: Parsley Root Veg Stew

Snack: Taro Chips

Day 29:

Breakfast: Spiced Hummus Avocado Toast

Lunch: Pork Loins with Leeks

Dinner: Chickpea Salad Wrap

Snack: Spiced Mango Trail Mix

Day 30:

Breakfast: Healthy Hot Multigrains Bowl

Lunch: Green Pesto Pasta

Dinner: Rotisserie Chicken Noodle Soup

Snack: Thai Style Eggplant Dip

CONCLUSION

In conclusion, I would like to express my sincere gratitude to you, dear reader, for using the "No Gallbladder Diet Cookbook for Women" to start your journey towards a healthier and happier life. I hope that as you have turned through the pages of these healthy and nourishing recipes you have found comfort in the knowledge that you are not the only one dealing with the difficulties brought on by a gallbladder issue.

May this cookbook lead you to a satisfying resolution to your health issues. My heartfelt wishes are with you for a healthy and happy journey towards rejuvenation. Take a wholehearted approach to every recipe, understanding that each ingredient has been thoughtfully selected to promote your health and improve your cooking.

Remember that following this diet and adjusting to it is about more than simply fueling your body; it's also about nourishing your soul and living a long, healthy life. I hereby encourage you to embark on this adventure with tenacity and resolve. Every meal should be an occasion to celebrate your dedication to self-care and a reminder of your inner power.

May this cookbook empower you to take charge of your health and inspire you to live life to the fullest. I'm really grateful for being a part of your wellness journey. Here's to your health, happiness, and a future filled with endless possibilities!

My Little Request

Dear Reader,

Thanks for your purchase, hope you enjoyed reading.

Could you please take a few seconds to leave a positive feedback on this book?

It'll help reach more people and we can collectively live healthier lives.

Thank you.

BONUS: MEAL PLANNER JOURNAL

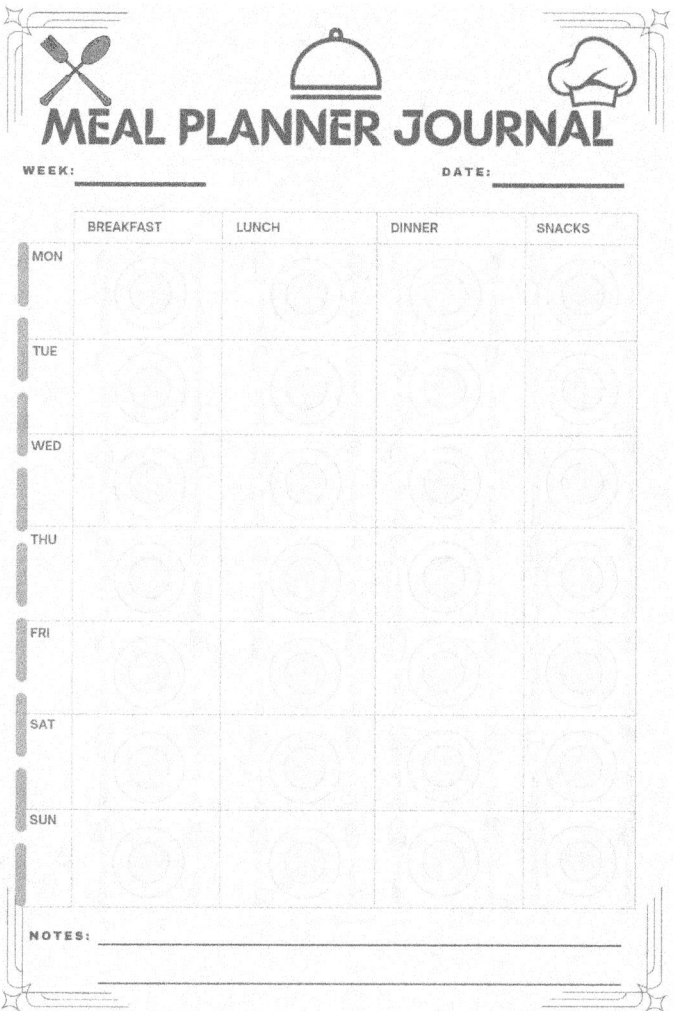

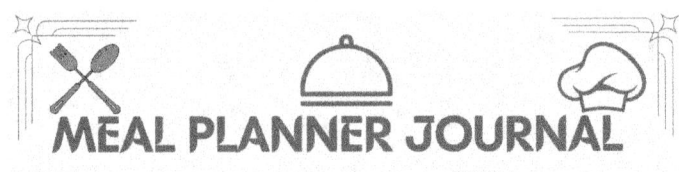

MEAL PLANNER JOURNAL

WEEK: _____   DATE: _____

	BREAKFAST	LUNCH	DINNER	SNACKS
MON				
TUE				
WED				
THU				
FRI				
SAT				
SUN				

NOTES: _____

_____

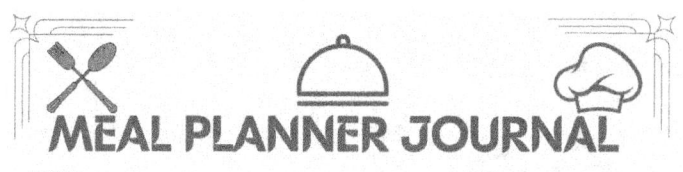

MEAL PLANNER JOURNAL

WEEK: _____   **DATE:** _____

	BREAKFAST	LUNCH	DINNER	SNACKS
MON				
TUE				
WED				
THU				
FRI				
SAT				
SUN				

NOTES: _____

_____

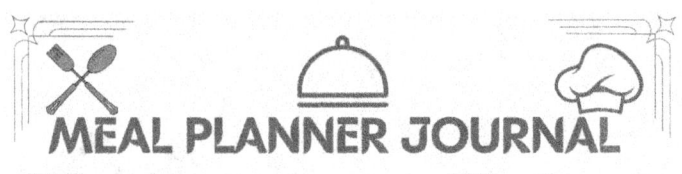

MEAL PLANNER JOURNAL

WEEK: _____   **DATE:** _____

	BREAKFAST	LUNCH	DINNER	SNACKS
MON				
TUE				
WED				
THU				
FRI				
SAT				
SUN				

NOTES: _____

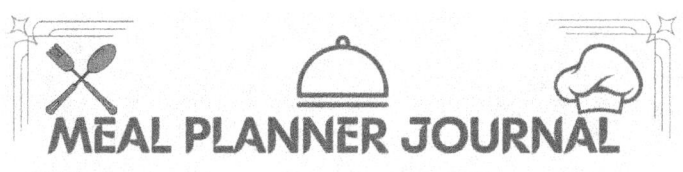

MEAL PLANNER JOURNAL

WEEK: _____   DATE: _____

	BREAKFAST	LUNCH	DINNER	SNACKS
MON				
TUE				
WED				
THU				
FRI				
SAT				
SUN				

NOTES: _____

_____

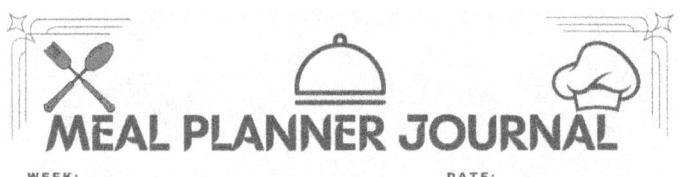

MEAL PLANNER JOURNAL

WEEK: _____   DATE: _____

	BREAKFAST	LUNCH	DINNER	SNACKS
MON				
TUE				
WED				
THU				
FRI				
SAT				
SUN				

NOTES: _____

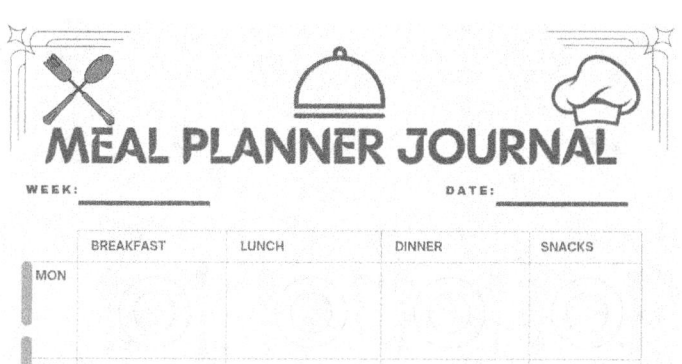

MEAL PLANNER JOURNAL

WEEK: _____   DATE: _____

	BREAKFAST	LUNCH	DINNER	SNACKS
MON				
TUE				
WED				
THU				
FRI				
SAT				
SUN				

NOTES: _____

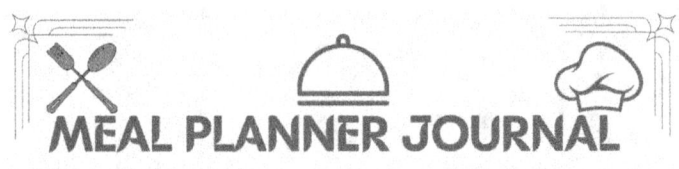

MEAL PLANNER JOURNAL

WEEK: _____   **DATE:** _____

	BREAKFAST	LUNCH	DINNER	SNACKS
MON				
TUE				
WED				
THU				
FRI				
SAT				
SUN				

NOTES: _____

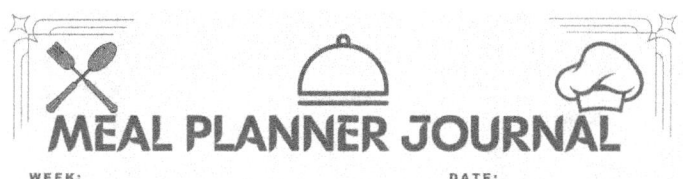

MEAL PLANNER JOURNAL

WEEK: _____   DATE: _____

	BREAKFAST	LUNCH	DINNER	SNACKS
MON				
TUE				
WED				
THU				
FRI				
SAT				
SUN				

NOTES: _____

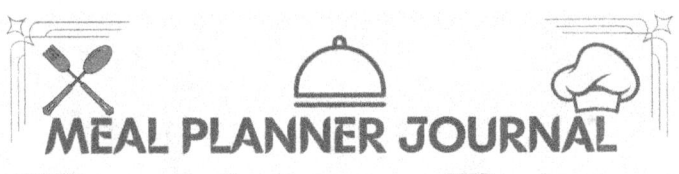

MEAL PLANNER JOURNAL

WEEK: _____   DATE: _____

	BREAKFAST	LUNCH	DINNER	SNACKS
MON				
TUE				
WED				
THU				
FRI				
SAT				
SUN				

NOTES: _____
_____

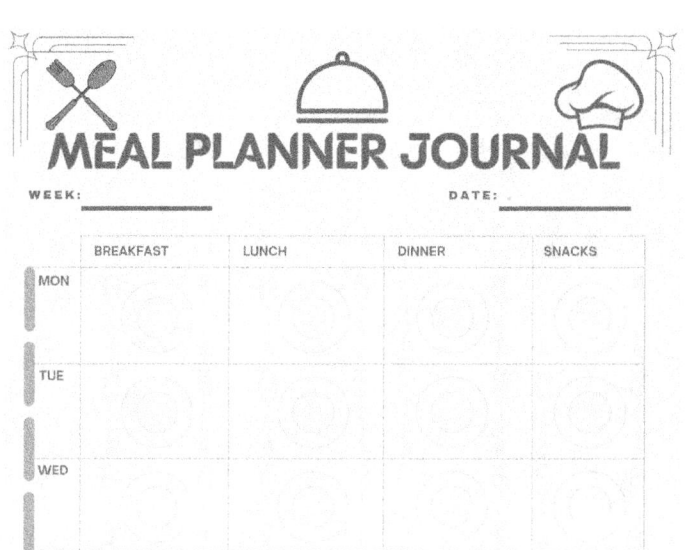

MEAL PLANNER JOURNAL

WEEK: _____   DATE: _____

	BREAKFAST	LUNCH	DINNER	SNACKS
MON				
TUE				
WED				
THU				
FRI				
SAT				
SUN				

NOTES: _____

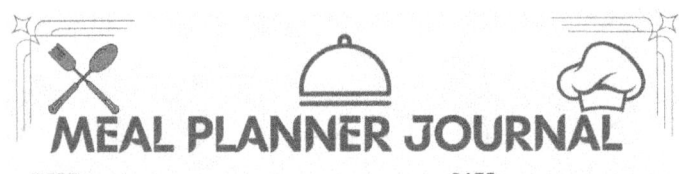

MEAL PLANNER JOURNAL

WEEK: _____   **DATE:** _____

	BREAKFAST	LUNCH	DINNER	SNACKS
MON				
TUE				
WED				
THU				
FRI				
SAT				
SUN				

NOTES: _____

_____

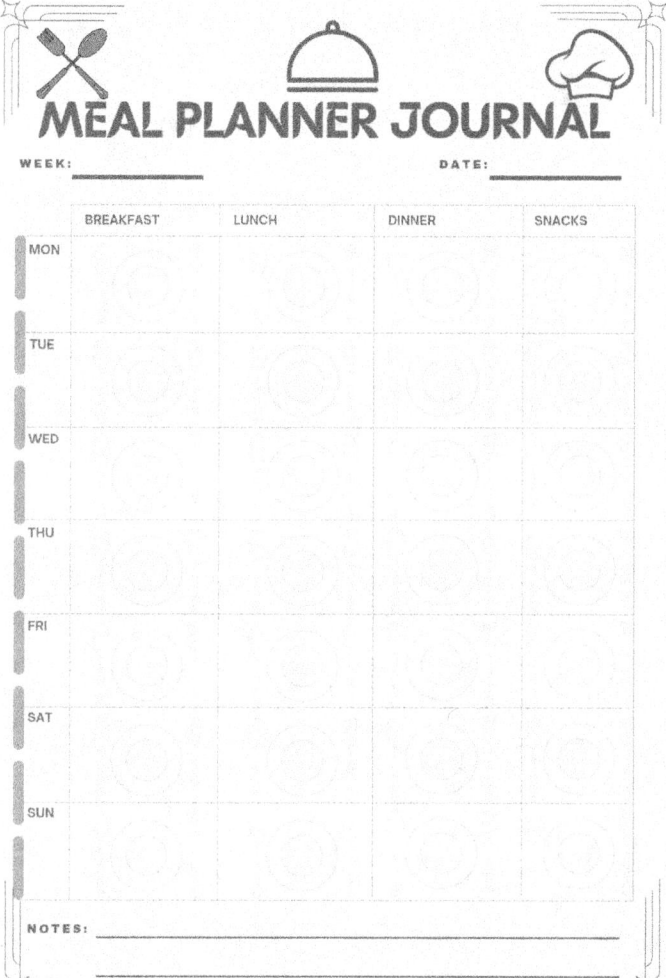

MEAL PLANNER JOURNAL

WEEK: _____   DATE: _____

	BREAKFAST	LUNCH	DINNER	SNACKS
MON				
TUE				
WED				
THU				
FRI				
SAT				
SUN				

NOTES: _____
_____

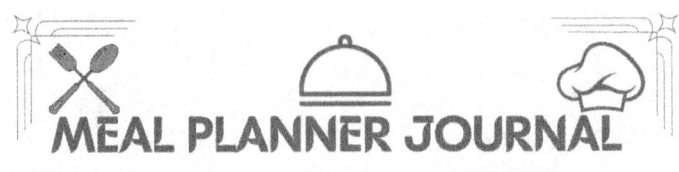

MEAL PLANNER JOURNAL

WEEK: _____   **DATE:** _____

	BREAKFAST	LUNCH	DINNER	SNACKS
MON				
TUE				
WED				
THU				
FRI				
SAT				
SUN				

NOTES: _____

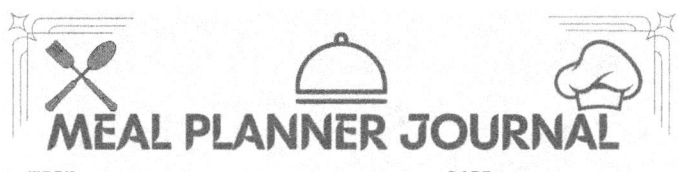

MEAL PLANNER JOURNAL

WEEK: _____   DATE: _____

	BREAKFAST	LUNCH	DINNER	SNACKS
MON				
TUE				
WED				
THU				
FRI				
SAT				
SUN				

NOTES: _____

_____

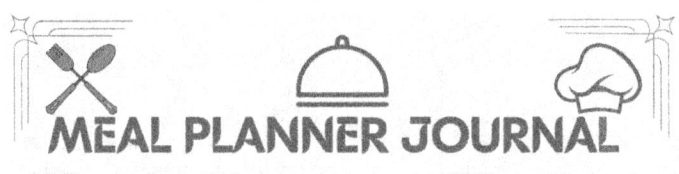

MEAL PLANNER JOURNAL

WEEK: _____   DATE: _____

	BREAKFAST	LUNCH	DINNER	SNACKS
MON				
TUE				
WED				
THU				
FRI				
SAT				
SUN				

NOTES: _____

_____

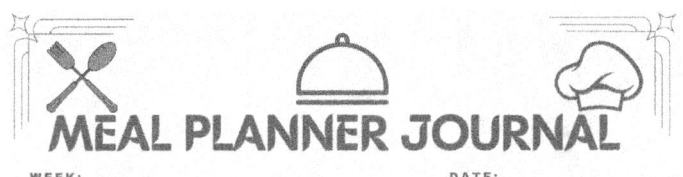

MEAL PLANNER JOURNAL

WEEK: _____   DATE: _____

	BREAKFAST	LUNCH	DINNER	SNACKS
MON				
TUE				
WED				
THU				
FRI				
SAT				
SUN				

NOTES: _____

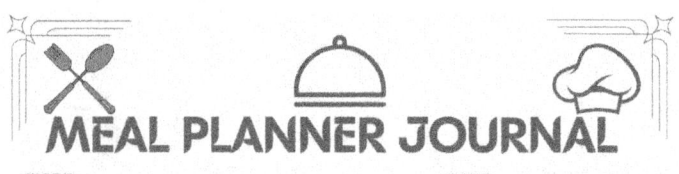

MEAL PLANNER JOURNAL

WEEK: _____   DATE: _____

	BREAKFAST	LUNCH	DINNER	SNACKS
MON				
TUE				
WED				
THU				
FRI				
SAT				
SUN				

NOTES: _____

_____

MEAL PLANNER JOURNAL

WEEK: _____   **DATE:** _____

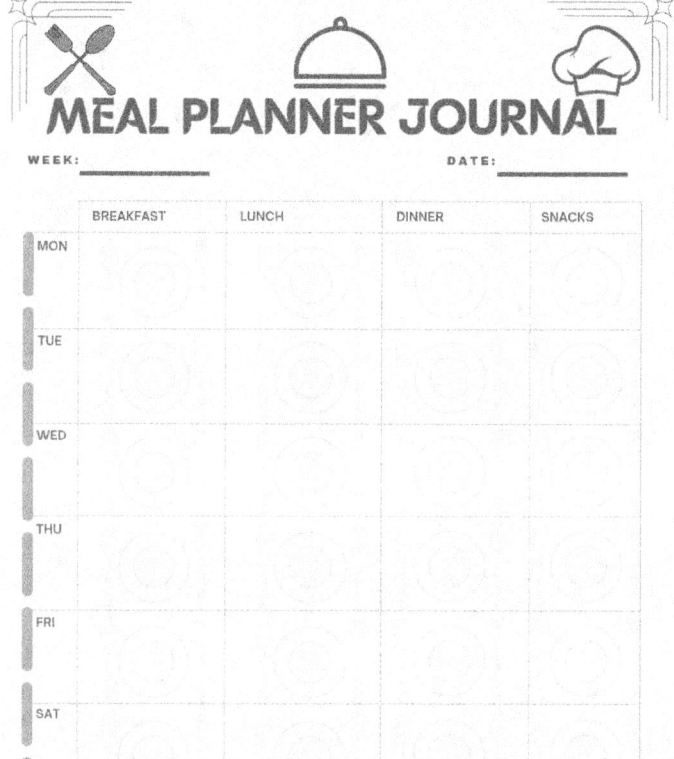

	BREAKFAST	LUNCH	DINNER	SNACKS
MON				
TUE				
WED				
THU				
FRI				
SAT				
SUN				

NOTES: _____

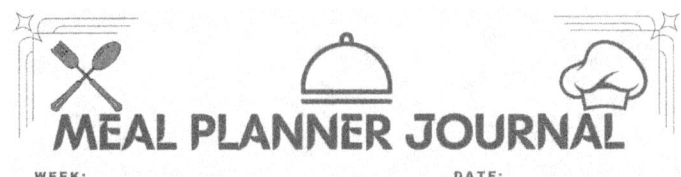

MEAL PLANNER JOURNAL

WEEK: _____   **DATE:** _____

	BREAKFAST	LUNCH	DINNER	SNACKS
MON				
TUE				
WED				
THU				
FRI				
SAT				
SUN				

NOTES: _____
_____

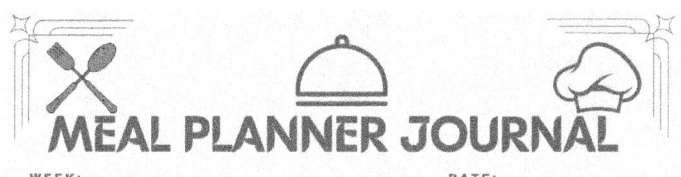

MEAL PLANNER JOURNAL

WEEK: _____   **DATE:** _____

	BREAKFAST	LUNCH	DINNER	SNACKS
MON				
TUE				
WED				
THU				
FRI				
SAT				
SUN				

NOTES: _____

_____